COLON CANCER

My Story

By

Anne Elizabeth Nixon

Text copyright © 2018

by Anne Elizabeth Nixon

All Rights Reserved

TABLE OF CONTENTS

Introduction – page 4

Digestive Tract – page 6

Attitude – page 7

Recognition & Tests – page 9

Physical Details – page 12

Newest Treatments – page 14

My History – page 17

Surgery – page 31

Ostomy Supplies – page 34

Pouches & Flanges – page 40

Recurrence – page 46

Complications – page 52

Odds & Ends – page 55

INTRODUCTION

The purpose of my book is to help you understand colon and colorectal cancer. It's something I know about from having had both myself, and having worked in the Tumor Clinic at the University of Oregon Medical School, now called OHSU.

First, the scientific definition of cancer: abnormal growth of cells that may invade or spread to other parts of the body.

While that is the technical description, it avoids mentioning the apprehension, confusion, and fear we have when we hear the word cancer. I want to tell you how you can do your best to prevent hearing the word cancer in regard to yourself; and if it should be, we'll discuss the treatment that is changing all the time. We have a better chance of survival these days with space-age technology to help us.

You'll also learn how your outlook is vitally important in returning to good health from cancer.

There are many diseases that necessitate removing part of the digestive tract, caused by various reasons. Adenocarcinoma (cancer) of the colon is a common one, with polyps often the beginning. Some people believe colon cancer is associated with diet, but most agree that family history is a more likely thread.

In my case, on my father's side I know of no cancers at all. But a great many of my mother's family died of cancer of the colon. I say "died" because cures were rare, and determining diseases were also. There were few cancer cures. The colonoscopy was developed in 1969 which began the start of prevention, no doubt.

To be a cancer survivor is a proud club. I am eternally grateful. But I can't claim to have been one who detected my tumor early, nor was it the reason for my survival. I wish I could—and because of my work experience with cancer, I should have. If you have a family history of colon cancer, be on the lookout for symptoms, which may include the following:

    changes in bowel habits
    alternating diarrhea and constipation
    rectal bleeding
    black, tarry stools (blood in stools)

DIGESTIVE TRACT

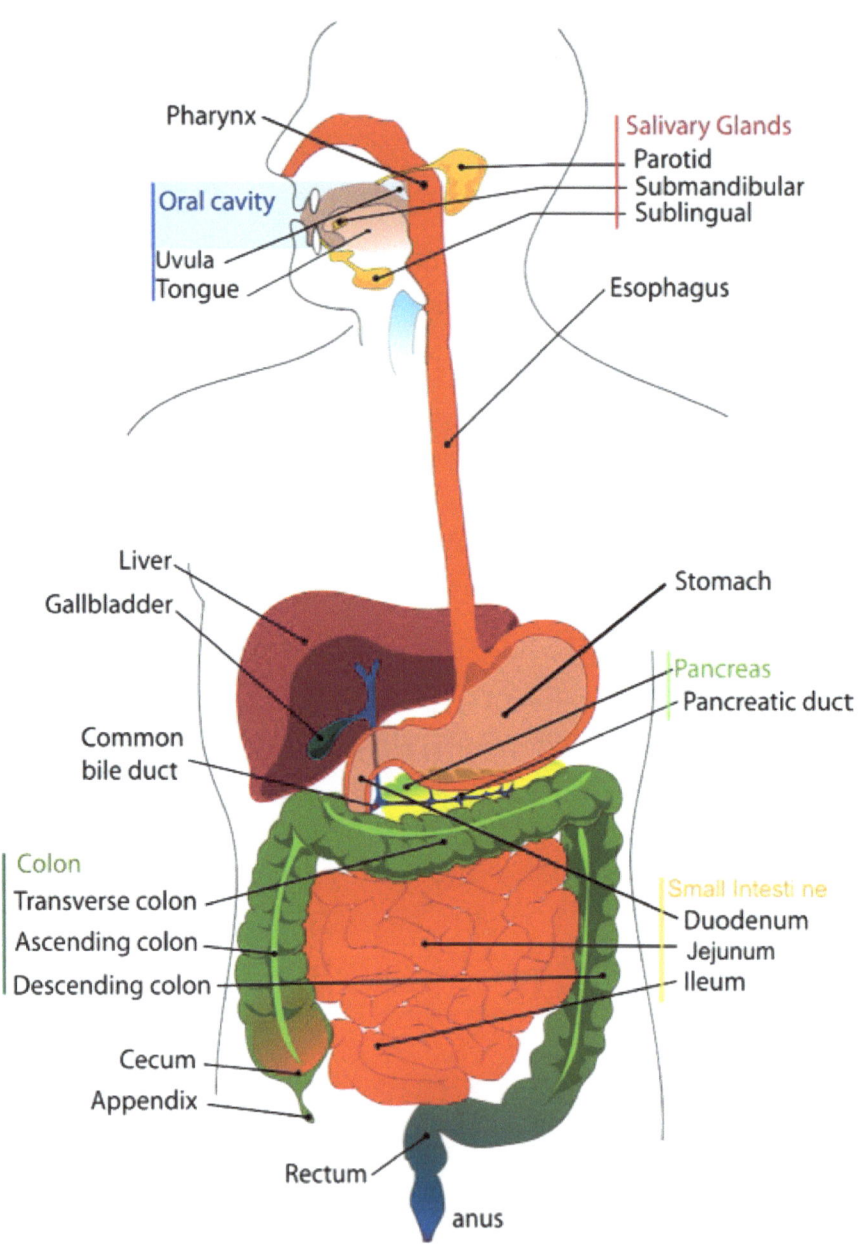

ATTITUDE

All of us have known negative people, those we prefer to steer clear of. But did we ever realize they may be their own worst enemy? They not only drive others away but may be hampering their health.

Thoughts—good, positive ones—are all-important. With colon cancer looming before me, I found myself thinking, "I'm going to beat this," over and over. I was born with an optimistic outlook, so possibly it was easier for me than others. But no matter how you feel toward life, a time of serious illness makes it necessary to try your best.

Positive thoughts and exercise stimulate <u>endorphins</u> in the body, which are chemicals that help to relieve pain or stress, and boost happiness.

If endorphins could be bottled for us we'd all have as much as we wanted or needed. But since we have to produce them ourselves, it's important we know about endorphins and how to increase them in our bodies.

Positive thoughts are the answer! And being as active as we can while fighting off disease is also important.

Keep yourself focused on killing that tumor, those nasty cells that are multiplying and want to do you harm. You don't want to produce hateful images, just powerful, positive ones. YOU are the powerhouse! Feel good about the strength you have been given by God or whatever power you believe in. Positive thinking is a healing force.

RECOGNITION & TESTS

Finding cancer at an early stage is vitally important, though some are almost impossible to discover at all, such as the pancreas. Men in particular often balk at a trip to the doctor's office, and others seldom admit a problem might exist. But at times just a routine visit will expose a symptom you might not have noticed. Answer your doctor's questions honestly, not what you think might be the right answer or one that doesn't suggest a problem. You will only hurt yourself.

One test for colon cancer is called Cologuard; you've probably seen it advertised on TV. Your doctor will, or should, include this test with a yearly physical exam. After opening a flat, square cardboard packet you are instructed to smear a bit of bowel movement, or feces, onto places in the area. Then you close it up and return it to your doctor to check for blood in your stool. While it is a good screening test, it's not absolutely positive, so you may need to have more tests.

Analyzing stool samples to find genetic changes associated with colorectal cancer is a new improvement. For that you are given a small plastic jar to return with stool inside. Be generous in your samples.

More specific exams are sigmoidoscopy and colonoscopy, where you cleanse your bowel, then the doctor sedates you before using a flexible scope to inspect your colon and rectum.

A barium enema x-ray may be helpful, as well as a CT scan of the abdomen, performed if your physician has reason to suspect a problem.

Polyps are important to be looked for; they are small growths on the wall of the colon, and may or may not be malignant. They can be found in other parts of the body but in the colon or rectum they are significant. At the time of a colonoscopy the doctor will remove them so they don't grow into cancerous growths.

If colon cancer runs in your family, you should take extra precautions. Ask your doctor at what age you should begin having a colonoscopy and how often.

And remember, requesting a second opinion if you aren't satisfied with a doctor's answers, is important. Don't hesitate to do so!

It may be that your tumor has spread to another organ or surrounding tissues. The term for that is **metastasis** for singular, or plural—**metastases**. Each cancer metastasizes (spreads) in certain ways to parts of the body.

Some go to the closest organs, and others can be spread farther away by the lymph channels or blood. You've heard of lymph nodes, a few being under your arms or in the neck or groin; they are for "catching" infection and disease so it doesn't travel on through your body.

PHYSICAL DETAILS

This first illustration is the large intestine which leads from the small intestine to the rectum.

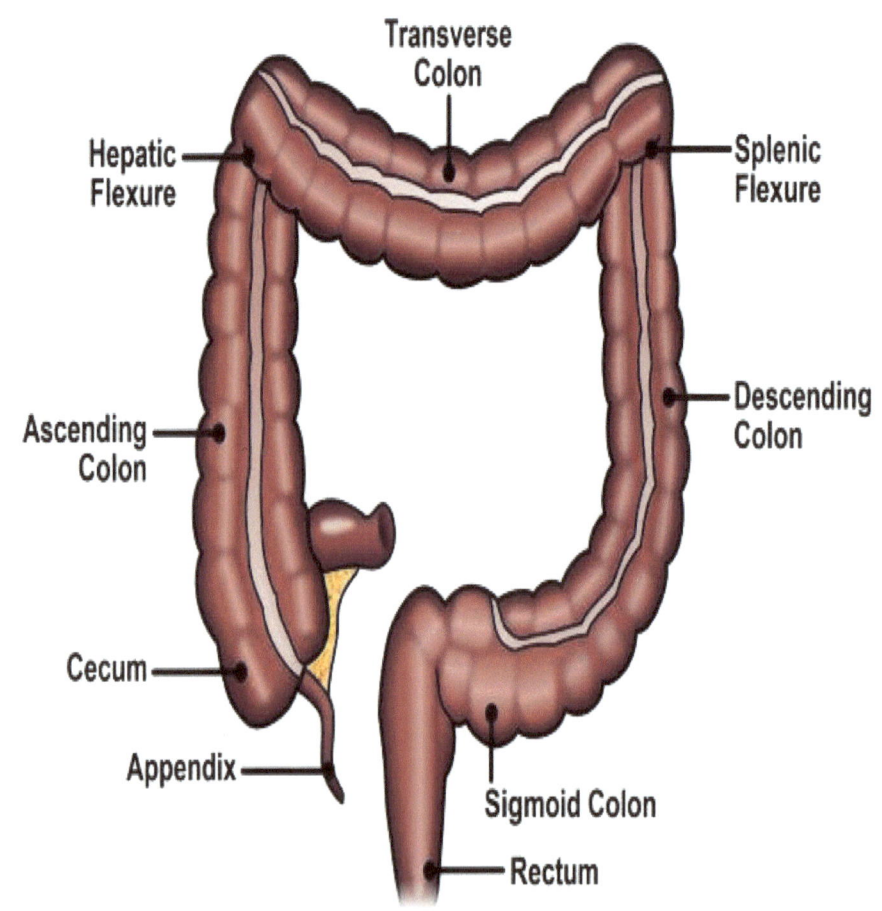

The next picture shows the entire colon, with the duodenum directly beyond the stomach. Marked portions that are lighter pink—duodenum, jejunum and ileum—make up the small intestine. The darker section is the large intestine.

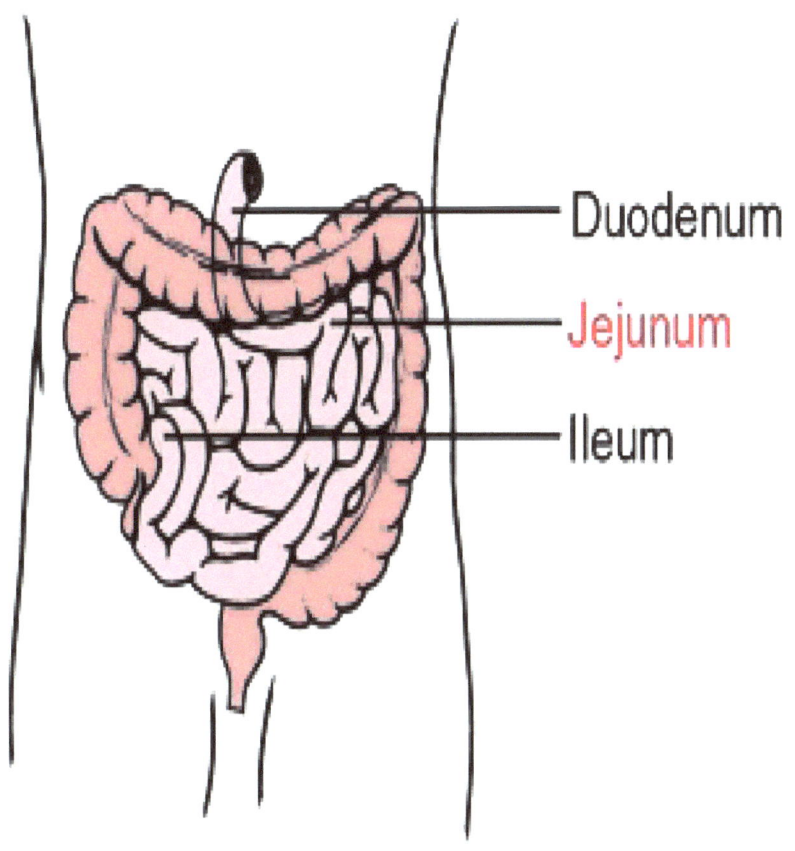

NEWEST TREATMENTS

Cancer research and therapy is at its finest. Among the most exotic is immunotherapy that has no side effects. Thinking back on my own chemotherapy, that seems unbelievable in the 17 years between now and then.

Immunotherapy is also called biologic therapy and is designed to boost our body's natural defenses to fight colon cancer. It uses materials made by the body or in a lab to improve, target or restore immune system function. Researchers have recently discovered a class of drugs targeting ways that tumor cells avoid the immune system. Those drugs are called checkpoint inhibitors. From there it gets too specific and scientific for us non-scientists. But it does seem like researchers may soon be on the way to discovering a way for our bodies to naturally fight cancer.

There are now tests to predict the risk of recurrent cancer. Various genes play important roles in the growth and spread of tumors. Doctors can more easily decide if chemotherapy should be used after treatment by using tests to identify these genes.

BRAF mutations are being studied for the spread of disease—metastases. (BRAF is a human gene that encodes a protein called B-raf.)

Recently chemotherapy has been treated by tablets—5-FU and other drugs. I personally know a lady being treated for breast cancer in both breasts by chemotherapy tablets; on one side the tumor has been found to disappear.

New drugs and chemotherapy are being tested, but most are available through clinical trials. Also, scientists are studying better ways to reduce symptoms and side effects and improve patients' comfort.

Imagine the great importance of these innovative discoveries! And they are just a few of the newest. Eventually it will be possible to enroll in a pilot study, but at this time it's very rare to impossible.

I've heard that terminal patients who want an experimental drug may be given a trial, but it is more likely not possible.

MY HISTORY

In telling you my story of colon cancer I hope to inspire you to get the best of care.

I was in charge of the Tumor Clinic at the University of Oregon Medical School from 1959 through 1964. My job entailed everything from setting up appointments, transcribing the doctors' dictation into charts (before computers), as well as running the Clinic and Tumor Board once a week.

Tumor Boards are invaluable meetings of medical doctors of all kinds—surgeons, pathologists, internists. They listen to a case being presented, examine the patient, then discuss their opinions for best treatment. Often ten or more doctors were gathered at ours, all volunteering their experience.

At the weekly clinic patients were first examined by a student (only male students then). When he finished he presented his findings to a physician. After that the doctor did an exam, they left the examining room, and talked about treatment for the patient. It gave the student education as well as giving a patient the advantage of his or her case being discussed. There were doctors on the staff at the Medical School as well as others who volunteered time there every Thursday morning. One drove in to Portland from the coast every week, and I admired him tremendously. There were many different types of cancer, and after I'd closed the clinic I began typing the words the doctors had dictated into a big, bulky "dictating machine"—which then, of course, was the latest in equipment. In that way I learned a great deal about the different kinds of cancer and what treatments were given. There were few innovative therapies in the early 1960s.

In about 1964 our residents (students who had become doctors, but not yet gone from the teaching / learning stage), were given the opportunity to begin the first Chemotherapy Clinic in Oregon. In a few examining rooms set aside for our resident, once a week this experimental treatment took place. After the doctor saw the patient he told me what drug to draw up into a syringe so he could administer the injection.

I will never forget the admiration I had for those patients, knowing they were part-taking in an unknown therapy that might end their lives sooner than without it, or if lucky, perhaps prolong them. But from past weeks, they knew the injection of chemotherapy that was so new and extremely strong, would incapacitate them with severe nausea and vomiting. I had never before realized in such stark terms the will to live, and I've never forgotten it.

My entire experience was overwhelming: working with doctors employed at the Medical School; doctors who donated their time to see patients in the Clinic and at Tumor Board; and the residents and interns in the University and County Hospital on campus. I've never felt that great pride in any job before or since.

To begin my colon cancer saga, I must admit to not going with my first instinct. One day I called my sister. "Have you been having any difference in your stools?" I asked like a newcomer to cancer symptoms. "Yes, I have," she replied, revealing they had been rather dark. (Mine was probably blood, while hers may have been what she'd been eating.) So I let it go instead of going to my doctor! Looking back on that, I see an act so foreign to me that I wonder if I really suspected something I didn't want to think about. Remember the children's parable about the ostrich who stuck his head in the sand? Well… Lesson #1

About the same time I had my every-10-year colonoscopy exam at a small rural hospital where we'd recently moved. The doctor was obviously foreign and I didn't know him, his history, or where he'd been educated. After the exam he told me I was free of any polyps or tumors, and I took him at his word.

Lesson #2: Find out the background of your doctor.

A year later when I discovered blood on my underclothes, I called for an appointment at that same Medical School where I had worked; and now I lived about 130 miles away from Portland, OR. I became the patient of a doctor I knew well, the "second in command" in the early 1960s when I had worked in the Tumor Clinic. He was an excellent doctor. This time I had sought the best I could find.
Lesson #3: Do research if necessary to get the best in that field.

"You have a tumor in the colorectal (lowest part of the bowel) area," he told me. I explained it hadn't been discovered on colonoscopy the previous year. We both realized that had been neglectful. Later when the doctor who had performed the colonoscopy and missed finding the tumor saw me, he patted my shoulder and assured me he'd perform my surgery. Not wanting to be rude, I let it go, but vowed I would never be seen by him again—for anything.
Lesson #4: Never go back to any medical personnel or doctor if you suspect the worst.

When I called OHSU, Oregon Health and Science University, where I had once worked, and asked for an appointment, I felt secure in the fact I'd be cared for by the finest.

After ordering and evaluating tests and x-rays, my doctor told me the findings—colorectal cancer, adding, "It would be best to have a colostomy, but it is your choice. Otherwise you will have no control of your bowels—because the tumor is so low in the rectum." He didn't have to wait long for my answer. "Yes," I told him. I definitely wanted the colostomy. In my case I knew all about them, but most patients need to be educated before being asked to choose. (A colostomy is a surgically-performed opening in your abdomen for evacuating your stools instead of through your anus.)

To determine whether it had spread to other areas of my body, including my liver, I was sent to have a PET scan. That was a new test at the time, only about 5 years old. After having an injection of radio-active material, I lay on a table while a machine picked up any areas of that radio-activity. I watched a screen (like a TV) give information to the technician in vivid colors. After it was over I asked the doctor if it had shown my liver free of tumor, and when he said, "No tumor in your liver," I happily told my husband, Don. It was a joyous moment!

Now it was time to begin treating my tumor, and I'd supposed that would mean surgery. But I was soon to learn there were new ways since I'd worked at the Medical School.

"You should have chemotherapy and radiation together before surgery," my doctor advised. "It will be five days a week for almost two months here at the University Hospital, but as an out-patient." He explained that would shrink my tumor, making the likelihood of a successful operation better.

My chemotherapy was one we'd used in our little experimental clinic years before, called 5-Fluorouricil, or 5-FU; it had been very successful. With a local anesthetic keeping me comfortable, a port, or entry point, was cut in my upper left chest and a tube inserted that led into a vein—called a Mediport. After the wound had healed, the chemo liquid would enter my body through that opening. It was important to be seen during that treatment, and since I was able to come to the clinic daily, I saw a nurse there. Some take their new pack of chemo home, then are visited by a nurse in a day or two.

Probably more common, a patient, along with others, sits in a special room at a hospital where chemotherapy slowly flows into the body. During that time he or she relaxes in an armchair for several hours. This is given in many time sequences, every other day, once a week, or whatever the doctors decide upon.

Mine was completely different from that. Each Monday I received a plastic pack of 5-FU; a bit of its contents would be pumped every 4 minutes through a tube which led to my port. The chemo pack was held in a black fabric bag with a belt that circled my waist. So as I dressed after taking a shower I put my clothes on over the tube that led from my chemo bag to my port. But the fanny pack always sat on my left hip outside my slacks or skirt. I learned to live with this bulky (approximately 4"x 6" x 2") pack, even in the shower, covered with a plastic bag; it would become simply the way I lived. It was all designed to be easy to wear.

Since I was to have my radiation each weekday morning at the Medical School, we decided to drive the 130 miles to Portland every Sunday afternoon and stay in town near the hospital until my treatments were over the following Friday, then drive home.

After locating a tiny apartment near the freeway which led to the medical complex, we left to find the nearest golf course. "I'll ride along with you whenever you want to play," I told Don enthusiastically. But I don't remember ever feeling well enough to go to the golf course, and I don't think Don went either. For chemotherapy to be strong enough to kill malignant cells, it must be debilitating, and I'd forgotten what I'd learned years before in that little chemo clinic I'd helped with, though I may have "forgotten" for a purpose—that of easing anxiety.

During the first week I felt normal; however, my body was being slammed with stronger chemicals and radiation therapy every seven days. As an example, Don used to drop me off at the hospital door where I walked to the chemo and radiation clinics, then he'd park the car. I'd make my way up the stairs, into an elevator, and find the treatment area. In a few weeks he left me off at the door, parked the car, and came back to go up with me, unsure if I could walk like I'd done before. When I was within 3 or 4 weeks from the end of therapy Don used valet parking, then got a wheelchair and pushed me upstairs.

The day of 9-11-2001, that infamous day when our United States was attacked, Don had helped me take a shower and I was sitting before the TV, waiting for him to be ready to get us some breakfast. (I didn't cook anymore.) I watched the plane slam into the first tower and, like everyone else, was shocked to think of the poor souls. I'd gone to tell Don about it, and when I got back to sit down, the second tower had begun crumbling. In my fragile state

I was unable to comprehend the enormity of it all. It took an hour or more for it to hit me.

To add to the shock, the night before I'd startled my husband with the news, "I can't take any more chemo and radiation." When Don heard that, he tried to convince me to continue, for it was to be my last week's treatment. But I was adamant. "I feel that I might die from another week of this." In some way I had an inner, sixth sense, that my body couldn't take any more, and I was fearful of that last week's highest dosage.

When we got to the clinic the TV was showing the horror of the attack and I burst into tears, completely out of control. A nurse led me to a quiet exam room to calm down, the room where I'd see the doctor and tell him my decision. He listened to me silently and I remember him telling me to think it over again, but whatever I wanted, he would agree to. Now I'd gone through two big happenings, my watching the attacks and telling the doctor of my decision. Through all of this, however, I had the support of a loving husband who, like the doctor, had gone along with my decision after I'd explained my reasoning .

That became the end of my pre-surgery therapy. We went back to our apartment, and while I lay on our bed, unable to help, Don loaded our belongings into the car. I couldn't do anything at all to help him, and it is a feeling that has stayed with me all these years. I had no energy to assist in any way; I was simply listless. As I said before, for the 5-FU to kill my tumor it must be very strong, and it had increased in strength each week.

Regarding the decision I'd made, listening to my body about stopping my therapies, may or may not have saved my life. The chemotherapy affects your brain as it does all the other parts, called "chemo-brain."

Now that I was at home it was time to recuperate and get strong enough for surgery. I remember how ineffective and strange I felt. "Come on, honey," Don urged, wanting desperately for me to eat. One day he was beside himself. "You'll die if you don't eat." Taking a plate of scrambled eggs he handed me, I tried, but couldn't get much down. It tasted rather metallic, but it wasn't that. It simply was impossible to eat. Those who have undergone chemo may have a similar story.

There are many nutritious drinks like Boost, Glucerna for diabetics, and others; I drank several of them daily to get the calories I needed for strength.

I'll bet you'd like a little humor here.

Don had a Russian Blue cat, a beautiful young fella that had jumped out of a cardboard packing box when a family moved in across the street from his parents, who we were visiting. Since that family had no idea where he belonged, had a dog or two, and didn't want him, Don wondered, "Shall we take him?" It took me only a moment to tell him, "Yes!"

That breed, which we discovered was a Russian Blue, is a one-person animal, and he adored Don but could barely tolerate me. However, after I finished my chemo and radiation, I lay on the couch every day for about a month, recovering before I had surgery. Sonovich (Don's Russian name for this rascal) jumped up and lay beside me every day, never leaving my side. He was a sweet, loving, gray kitty, and it made me feel good to have him there.

After having my surgery and leaving the couch for good. Sonovich, who had been my constant companion, returned to being Don's cat, turning a blind eye to me. He'd given me his "all," but now he was back to being his master's side-kick, riding on a wheelbarrow, chasing birds and mice, and all things boy kitties adore!

After about a month I was admitted to the hospital for surgery by the doctor I knew from my Tumor Clinic days. When you are treated at a teaching hospital it is routine that your care is shared by students, interns, residents and professors/doctors   . I found it very interesting as well as reassuring. My case would be discussed by them all, so I felt nothing was being missed. Surgery went well but I remember little of that time in the hospital. Before leaving I was instructed by an ostomy nurse how to care for my colostomy.

By the time I was home again and recuperating, I had lost 20 pounds. It seemed impossible to gain it back. A nurse one day advised, "Make a big sheet cake and put lots of frosting on it." I must have looked startled, for she grinned, probably wishing it were for her. "Then you should eat a piece for dessert after every meal, breakfast, lunch and dinner." I'm not one to enjoy frosting, so after a couple of meals topped off with my huge cake, I scraped off the thick top layer. But it worked. Soon I had gained my weight back.

It took several months to get bac k to feeling normal, but before long I was gardening and I began playing golf occasionally with Don. Eventually I joined the women's golf club and with them and Don, I played a couple of times a week. Later we added Saturday night dinner and dancing with friends. By then my colostomy didn't bother me in activities. However, it is something you must get used to.

Remember: When I worked in the Tumor Clinic there were no innovative therapies as I mentioned before. Chemotherapy had not become a treatment yet until I was about to leave. Nowadays we are so fortunate to have choices.

But still, the repositioning of the colon is as important as it has always been, for our bodies haven't changed! We still need a way to empty bowel contents like we did years ago, and for the foreseeable future.

When doctors remove part of the colon for any reason, it may be necessary to reposition it to empty from an opening in the abdomen rather than the rectum, called a colostomy. If it's to be permanent, the anus is closed by a surgical procedure, and from that time on the patient's bowel contents will flow through the new opening, called a stoma. While it might sound terrible to you as you first read this, think about it—your life has been saved and you will simply go to the bathroom in a different way. Thousands, millions of us have done this for years.

If the portion of the colon surgically removed is the ileum, an ileostomy would be the name of the exit point, still just another way to void waste, as with a colostomy. But because the ileum is closer to the stomach the excrement is more liquid.

Your doctor or a nurse will explain the way you should eat after colon surgery, about smaller portions and what foods to avoid. It's important to follow through on that for your future good health may depend upon it. Later you may be able to go back to your former habits, but again, maybe not. If you want a healthy, pain-free life, listen and follow that advice.

SURGERY

Your doctor may prefer surgery right away, depending on your tumor and whether it has metastasized (spread). There are a variety of ways to treat cancer, like chemo or radiation, but it could be both chemotherapy and radiation. Or it could be surgery only. At the time of mine in 2001, I believe not having surgery immediately may have been a new idea at the U of O medical school, but I'm not sure now.

Before your operation your bowel must be cleaned out as it was before a colonoscopy. I've heard people say they were admitted and had the cleansing as an in-patient. But that is an expensive way for both the hospital and patient unless you must come in the previous day for some reason.

Your stay may be up to one week or more. It's important to get out of bed as soon as they ask you to so you don't lose strength, something that was unheard of many years ago. But someone will help you walk at first, then you'll be reminded to do so yourself after feeling safe. It's an important step, and one to be proud of. Bring something comfortable to wear home as your abdomen will be tender.

Non-invasive surgery is the latest in surgical procedures. Laparoscopy allows your surgeon to perform your operation through an ultra-small incision. You will discover you have a great deal less pain later, a plus to be sure. My colorectal surgery scar from 2001 is no doubt longer than many nowadays. But when you have a previous incision the doctor may want to use the scalpel on part or all of that scar. If you're interested, don't hesitate to ask about your procedure ahead of time.

    Prior to surgery you will be given a hospital gown or whatever you're to wear, and you'll try to get comfortable on a gurney. Then an aide will begin checking your blood pressure and temperature and take an EKG, leaving you hooked up. When a nurse gets an IV started as well as a catheter you'll know it won't be long before you're headed for the operating room. This is all done so you'll be ready when the time comes. Your anesthesiologist will want to talk with you to find out if there are any red flags, anything you're allergic to or has given you a problem during prior surgeries. Are you drug sensitive? If so, be sure to tell him or her, for that might be extremely important—it was for me once. Think carefully about bad reactions you may have had. Occasionally these questions will have been done several days before you enter the hospital.

Soon you'll be wheeled into a room that looks foreign to you, full of sterile equipment. As the intravenous (IV) anesthetic begins entering your body you will begin viewing the area through a fuzzy haze, then you'll remember nothing until you come to and it's all over. It will take time for you to waken, and that will be in what's appropriately called the Recovery Room. Eventually you'll feel like you just had a nap, but you'll discover you're hooked up to a BP cuff on your arm, and other gadgets which personnel will be monitoring.

Hospital costs are high, and for a little levity, I'll tell you what my mother said one day many years ago. Having just come home from the hospital, (when they kept you there, in bed, until you were weak), she moaned, "Thirty-three dollars a day! Where will it ever end?!"

If you have reason to believe you may have serious illnesses, choose a Supplemental Insurance that will give you the most coverage you can afford. You probably won't regret it.

OSTOMY SUPPLIES

If you don't need a colostomy, this section may not be of interest to you. However, many of us know someone who has a colostomy which would give us information we might appreciate.

An ostomy is simply a way for waste to leave the body through a stoma, and stored until emptied, in a pouch. We are discussing the colon and ileum, but there is also a urostomy for the urinary tract. Other diseases than cancer can be reasons for ostomies, either temporary or permanent. If temporary, a second surgery is necessary for reconnecting the two ends of whatever organ has been severed; this is called anastomosis.

Before going to surgery, an ostomy nurse came into my room. "I'd like you to sit on the side of the bed," she began, patting the sheet. She felt my abdomen and said, "I'm marking the place so the surgeon will know where to put the opening of your bowel." Then, with a felt pen, she placed an X in the spot where my abdomen was smooth and didn't have a crease. At the time I had only an inkling of what she was talking about, for while I'd worked with patients who had colostomies, I'd never actually seen one. You might have a general idea, too, but everything will be new and strange to you. That's to be expected. The reason the nurse made the decision was because in surgery I would be lying flat and the surgeon would not know where on my tummy to place the stoma.

After my operation the same nurse returned to demonstrate how a flange would be applied to my abdominal skin around the stoma. "This is what you'll be using every day," she explained, smiling. "And this," she said, holding up what I learned was a pouch, "fits onto it."

A **flange,** that adheres to your skin, is a round or rectangular piece of strong material with a circular hole in the center that fits around your stoma, the new opening of your bowel. A plastic ring on that flange attaches to another ring on a pouch, holding the two together.

A **pouch** is a small bag that fits onto that flange. As you wear it, it will fill with bowel contents, or feces; some pouches are closed-ended and others open-ended. I personally use the closed end; when it fills I just take it off and replace it with another pouch. You must be careful to change it only when it's full or mostly full though, for if you have Medicare you are allowed only a certain number for each 3-month period. If you are paying for all supplies you must think of the cost.

And speaking of cost, there are choices to make: the open-ended pouches will last longer than closed-ended ones; clear, see-through pouch material is less expensive than opaque fabric. Since it will never be seen by other than those closest to you, it may not matter. You can also choose a pouch with a filter for odor, though there is fluid you can order to counteract any odor. When you begin ordering you can make choices. And don't hesitate to ask questions about features and cost as you begin placing orders; they are very knowledgeable and can answer any questions you might have.

There are many different companies to choose from; personally, I think it's easier to buy all supplies from one; they will bill your insurance and if you need something again you won't have to wonder where it came from. When you get home from the hospital you will probably be given samples and perhaps the names of companies to call that sell colostomy and ileostomy supplies.

Companies selling ostomy supplies: Liberator, Edgepark, Smith & Nephew, Bard, Marlen and others. They sell all kinds of medical supplies, though we're only interested in ostomy equipment. A few of the **best-known brands are**: Coloplast, Hollister, Convatec for example. I order my supplies from a large company in the northeast U.S., but a friend gets hers from a smaller one in a neighboring city. Each company has a catalogue with the supplies you'll need, giving you pictures, explanations, sizes and product numbers. The supply companies are always happy to send you free samples; I've gotten them many times. It may be of no help or possibly solve a big problem. Never hesitate to ask. While I'm on hold I hear a voice telling of the newest products. When something interests me I ask for a sample or order one to try.

If you have medical insurance it may help with the expense. Medicare pays part and Medicaid will likely pay.

Because there are many "styles" of equipment, I suggest you begin with a small, one-month order at first; then when you find what you prefer, order the 3-month supply if you want.

Not all ostomy supplies will be the same. The closures for **open-ended** pouches in particular, will be different. (See pictures in the next chapter.) From pictures in a catalogue you can decide which you'd like to try.

And depending on the protrusion of your stoma, you will have to get the **flange** that "fits." Your doctor or ostomy nurse can tell you what you have. For stomas that don't protrude you'll need a convex flange, and for ones that do protrude, the more level flange is best for you.

If **one-piece units** are more to your liking—flange and pouch together in one piece, try a sample of that, but I'd suggest you begin with a 2-piece. Ask the ostomy nurse to tell you what size your stoma is so as to know what size opening in the flange you'll need. There are many sizes and shapes of stomas, and the nurse will measure yours and tell you what you should order in the future; if yours is oval you have the choice of cutting the opening yourself with special scissors you can order from the company,

For an **irregularly-shaped stoma** you can order soft, stretchable rings called barrier rings. They can help keep from having leakage around the edges, as well as if the abdomen around your stoma has highs and lows it will help equalize the level. That sounds very complicated, and it may be at first, but when you discover what suits you and feels right, you can order the same thing each time. If in doubt, order a sample.

Your stoma may change over time, and you can ask your supplier for a paper with cut-outs for measuring your stoma—or one may come in the catalogue. By holding the cut-out openings over your stoma, the correct size for an opening will be evident, and you can order that size.

As I mentioned previously, for open-ended pouches you can buy a liquid deodorant from supplier that you add when first putting it on, and can be added each time it's emptied.

POUCHES & FLANGES:

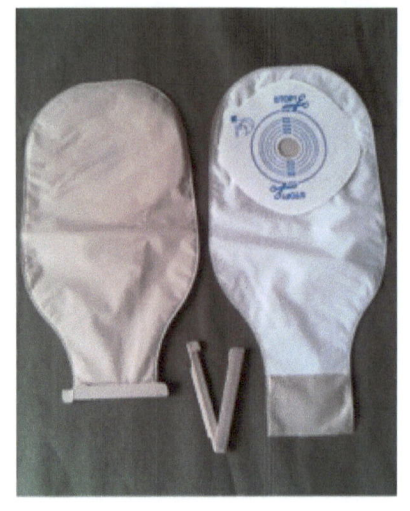
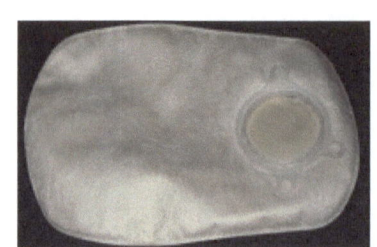
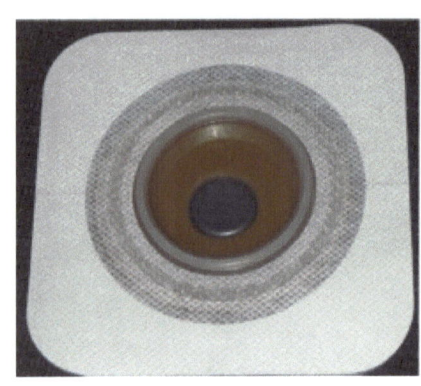

Top Left: One-piece, open-ended pouches. (There are also closed end, one-piece.)
Top Right: Closed-end pouch that fits onto a flange. (Also in open-ended.)
Bottom left: Flange. This one is convex. (For a flat stoma.)

The flange ring and pouch ring must fit– flat or convex.

In the left picture is the one-piece outer side, and on right is one-piece showing the built-in flange that goes against your skin. After using scissors to cut a hole for the correct size of your stoma (see the lines around the center) you'd peel off the paper and flatten it against your abdomen, with hole over your stoma. The "glue" would hold it in place. The V-shaped object is closure for drain end, though some have built-in closures.

Emptying your open-ended pouch: When you empty your open-ended pouch sit on the toilet and unlock the bottom end. On some there is a plastic piece that clamps over that (see above pictures) and others have a Velcro piece so that after folding it over a few times the Velcro piece holds it tightly. Using fingers, work feces down and out the opening. Use toilet paper to wipe several times, then close. If using liquid deodorant, put it in now before closing. You will probably have to squeeze it to make it round and open enough to clean and add deodorant.

Abdominal hernia: A few years after my surgery I noticed my abdomen needed more and more "fixing" with the soft, sticky barrier rings to make the field level. It hadn't been that way previously, and I had occasional leaking accidents. When I called the ostomy supply company to ask questions I discovered I could order a 1-inch wide elastic belt that hooked onto each side of my flange. On one end it could be made longer or shorter to fit the size of my tummy.

That worked for a while, but then I discovered the reason for my discrepancy: I had an abdominal hernia that was adjacent to my stoma. What that means is the muscles and tissues of my abdomen had a tear and a small pocket of my abdomen was coming through that tear. I could push it back in at first, but then pressure enlarged the tear and it became harder to manage. The doctor helped me understand all that, and I began wearing a wide mesh belt with a circular hole at one end, allowing the colostomy pouch to be brought through. At the other end is a wide Velcro closure. The belts can be ordered through your ostomy company, but measure the diameter of the raised circle of flange opening because the round hole in the belt must fit around that without being too small (tight) or too large (loose). The belts can be mesh or a smooth fabric, and I have used both over the years. In hot weather I prefer the mesh, but the fabric one has no lines that might show through light slacks or skirts. **See hernia belt.**

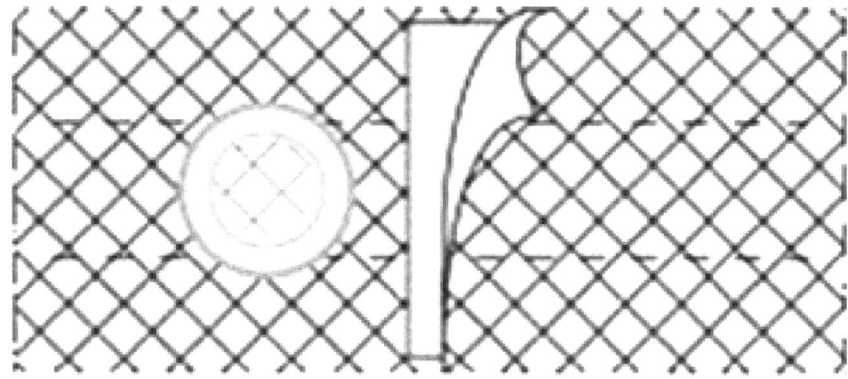

They will be listed and pictured in the ostomy catalogue, and without insurance they are $90 or a bit more, but Medicare pays part and insurance may also. Whether you get help paying for the belt to keep your hernia secure, it is vital that either you wear the belt or have surgery for repair. Nu-Hope, the manufacturer of these, has a website and offers a $20 discount, and lists the measurements for openings. For the first-timer it's worth looking it up online.

If this is not clear, let me try to explain: you must measure the diameter of what will be pushed through the hole in the mesh belt. Pull up your pouch so you can see that ring on flange. With a ruler, take the number of inches from one side to the other and that's the size of hole to be ordered in mesh belt.

You may say, "Whew, this is too complicated for me!" It may seem so now, but you'll have help before leaving the hospital, and the supply company personnel can answer questions for you. Don't hesitate to take advantage of their help.

It might be a good idea to request a catalogue for ostomy supplies before your surgery. The easiest way to get a list of all the suppliers is to go online and Google "ostomy supply companies." After you begin ordering your flanges and pouches you can get samples sent to you, but don't depend upon them arriving right away. A regular order will come more quickly. And don't forget, the companies will bill your insurance at no extra cost.

There's no question that a colostomy is a learning experience. You'll make mistakes like I did, but go on to try something else. Eventually you'll say, "This is a snap!" like I do. I've spent 17 years at this—trust me.

One thing I've discovered is how uncomfortable constipation is for anyone with a colostomy. Diarrhea is inconvenient, and will no doubt keep you close to your supplies, but the discomfort in your abdomen is often debilitating with constipation. If you tend that way, think about whether you drink enough water every day. With a "yes" answer, adding fiber mixed in a full glass of water every day may help you. Or a bran cereal each morning may do the trick. Whatever it takes, you will be much more comfortable if you think about this before your operation and get the supplies.

Note: Don't take any fiber additive immediately after surgery. Ask your doctor when you might begin, if it's necessary to use it.

RECURRENCE

My recurrence began in an extremely unusual way. From absence of even dizziness in my life I had an attack of what was thought to be vertigo and twice was taken to the Emergency Room. When asked if I saw the room spinning, I always replied, "No, it's lurching, not spinning." But to get up out of my chair I needed two people for help.

By chance I had a follow-up appointment with my cardiologist who noticed I was severely anemic, and determined it was important to find out what was the cause. In the interim he started me on ferrous sulfate, or iron tablets, to curb my anemia.

He and my primary care doctor sent me to one who performs endoscopies (a tube inserted into your throat down to the stomach—after being sedated). He discovered multiple stomach and esophageal bleeding ulcers, but was aware they were not large enough to cause the blood loss I was experiencing. So after a prep to make me have diarrhea for cleansing, I was again sedated and he examined my bowel (and in my case not through my rectum but through my colostomy). It was then he found the large bleeding tumor in my ascending colon. After taking pictures and biopsies (snipping out pieces of tissue to send to the pathology lab), he removed the scope. I remember how surprised I was to have another cancerous tumor after all the years since my first one—17 years.

Not directly related to my tumor, but related in a roundabout way, when my severe anemia was lessened by the iron tablets, I never had a bout of "vertigo" again. Evidently it was the loss of blood from my cancerous colon tumor that caused my lurching dizziness.

CT scans helped the doctor understand what should be done. But until the pathologist's report gave the exact type and whether it was a metastasis (spread), there was not a clear answer to that question.

I have a pacemaker, and if you have one too, you're probably aware you cannot have an MRI due to the fact that it is magnetic. That's why I have had CT scans while you may be scheduled for MRIs.

It was obvious I'd need surgery, and while I could be admitted sooner at a local hospital, my operation was going to be too involved for that one. UCSF, the University of California at San Francisco, was what I needed. After finding I could register myself I called and got set up, though most people are referred by a doctor. Before long I was contacted and was given an appointment to see my surgeon.

My son took me, and had the advantage of hearing what the doctor planned and could ask questions himself. From there they sent me to the anesthesiology department and I answered questions about my past surgeries and anesthesia. If you must drive a considerable distance as I did, it's best to get as many things accomplished in one visit as possible.

From that time on it was a matter of waiting until they had a time slot for me, and the date was changed several times.

The following is a very precise explanation of pathology being determined during an operation at the Mayo Clinic. The University of California at San Francisco (UCSF) does the same, as well as OHSU, the university hospital in Portland, OR. Few others are as sophisticated.

Beginning of article: Mayo Clinic is one of the few medical centers in the nation to use a tissue freezing process for analyzing operating room tissue samples on a routine basis. The process allows pathologists to rapidly analyze and diagnose tissue samples while the patient is still in the operating room. The rapid turn-around of results saves patients time and money, since one surgery at Mayo can take the place of two or three procedures at other institutions.

During an operation, tissue is transferred to the frozen tissue lab directly from the operating room. There, it is placed on a freezing microtome machine where the bottom of the sample is frozen within seconds. A razor-thin slice of tissue is extracted from the frozen section, prepared on a slide and placed under the microscope for review. In many other medical centers, this process takes at least 24 hours to complete.

After reviewing the sample, the pathologist conveys the test results to the surgeon in the operating room. Immediately, the Mayo Clinic surgeon can adjust the operation accordingly and avoid unnecessary re-operations.

End of article.

I was told my surgery would probably take about 4 hours and I should expect to be in the hospital one week.

Finally the date arrived. I was in a teaching hospital as I was in 2001, and before the procedure began I was given the opportunity to be in a study regarding pain suppression, which I chose to take part in. A hair-like needle was inserted into my spine for anesthesia to be administered. During the days that was in place I had no pain whatsoever; a medical young student came by daily to get information from me about how I felt. I had only pleasant words for him, for it was wonderful. I must stress that you are never pressured to take part in any study, and I encourage you to make up your mind and not feel it's something you "should" do.

A team of doctors and students checked on me daily, making rounds twice a day. They gave me results of lab work that was done every morning at 5 AM, and any x-rays, some with a portable machine. I came to know the team and looked forward to hearing about my progress.

When you have pain in the hospital, don't hesitate to take whatever medication the doctor offers. Your discomfort will diminish as time goes on, and the drugs prescribed will then be less strong.

Years ago I had trouble eating after my first chemotherapy, and again this time after my surgery. You may or may not experience this, but if food tastes good to you, eat to keep your strength up. I lost weight again, and finally, when I got home, decided to forget about trying to gain the 13 or so pounds back. I became active and felt if I was a bit less weight, so be it. Eating desserts puts on weight, but a well-rounded diet is always best. If you are diabetic, talk to your doctor before trying to get back to normal weight with sweets.

You must be careful not to overdo, but walking and light exercise are important to get your strength back again. If you are sent to rehab for a few weeks after being in the hospital, you will no doubt have physical therapy. I found that very helpful, and until strong enough to be dismissed by their nurse, I had biweekly visits. That private company I chose from a list provided by Medicare. There are many in every city.

During the time you are in rehab or having physical therapy all medical supplies must be ordered through the physical therapists. In my case all my previous colostomy supplies that I ordered myself, have to be gotten that way. Unfortunately, no one told me until I was a bit low on pouches.

If you need supplies of any kind, talk to your physical therapy nurse or other employee and get them ordered. As I say, they are the ONLY ones who can order anything for you. The reason is because Medicare is paying for them and that's their way of being in control of the situation.

COMPLICATIONS

In my first chapter I explained how important it is to keep your spirits up. While it is, there may be times when it seems impossible. I found that true during my second colon cancer recovery. The surgery was very complicated, and food would not travel a short distance from the surgery to my stoma because of numerous adhesions, swelling and other problems.

One morning when this happened I began vomiting because nothing could get through; a bit of that vomit got into one lung. That produced aspiration pneumonia, which was a serious set-back, and I was started on antibiotics. Each morning a portable x-ray machine was wheeled into my room so my team could follow my progress.

Not long after that I had heart failure due to some heart issues I've had in the past. That had to be treated in another of UCSF's hospitals across San Francisco, so I was taken by ambulance there. That not only changed my treatment but added to my length of stay.

Next was a second bout of pneumonia, not from having gotten vomit in my lung this time. I was moved to another floor and antibiotics begun again.

When my doctors asked about pain and other questions each time they visited me, I occasionally told them how discouraged I'd become. They understood, for my stay, from five days, had stretched into weeks. Encouraging me to eat was part of their daily routine. Luckily, I discovered "berry/banana shakes" and drank two or more of those each day. While they didn't put on any weight, they were nutritious.

One morning my team came by with news that threw me into my happiest moments for weeks—I would go home that day! It's hard for you to imagine how elated I became, for it had been one month and one day! And during that time I'd had no shower or shampoo, so they promised me those. I'd never even seen the inside of my bathroom, for by this time I had a permanent catheter. And I'd been transferred to different floors that specialized in the type of problem I had at the time.

When it was time to leave I happily told them all good-bye, and headed by wheelchair to the front door. The San Francisco hospital had arranged for my transport, and the driver wound about city streets until we got to the freeway leading north. Then, for a special treat, he took a back, winding road part of the way so I could see cow pastures, rolling hills and beautiful orchards. It was bouncy but I was thrilled. He let me off at the rehab center where I would spend about ten days recuperating. Then I was picked up by the driver of my assisted care home, to return to my apartment, my good friends—and my Tom (cat). I'd missed them for all that time, but especially Tom who had been cared for by loving friends, both his and mine! What a thrilling moment to be back!

ODDS & ENDS

If you know you are going to be in the hospital it's wise to plan ahead. I won't go into children, for that is very personal and obvious. Pets need care, whether it be by a friend or relative, or a professional. It's always preferable to let an animal stay in its own surroundings, especially when its main source of love will be gone. But leaving any animal unattended is unthinkable. I'm sure you'll agree with me.

While plants are not in the same category, they may need watering occasionally, and getting someone to come in or water outdoor flowers will ease your mind if you'll be gone that long. Like I discovered, you are never sure how long you'll be away.

If you are a computer person you will understand this next idea, but if not, just ask a friend to phone your pals to let them know how you are. However, if you have a computer and "do" email, this should be easy to understand: before I went into the hospital for my colon cancer surgery I emailed my good friends. Then I asked my son to email those same friends and relatives after my surgery and occasionally after that. I passed on to him my email of friends, so all he had to do was bring up my "master plan of addresses" and begin his message. It was simple and eased the minds of those I cared about and who cared about me and my well-being. If you don't have anyone who can do that, you might call or email pals before being admitted, to tell them you'll be in the hospital and for what reason, adding the length of time you expect to be there. You can save the addresses and get off a short message when you get home.

Don't overdo after your surgery! Even after going to rehab for ten days I had to find out the hard way. At my assisted care home I always played bocce ball, and while it's not strenuous, after an abdominal operation it is. So, for several weeks I did nothing but watch others play. And I rested and slept in my nice easy chair a great deal of every day except to go to the dining room for meals.

But one Saturday my family asked me over for dinner; they picked me up and returned me—which seemed simple enough. But the next day I realized I'd been foolish to go anywhere so soon. It had been too much, and too soon! Err on the side of over-indulgence to yourself. Be extra careful about lifting, eating foods too spicy or eating too much at one time, getting too little sleep, and beginning your regular routine too quickly. If you have any bending over, like my Tom's litter box, get someone to do it for you for a while. There are many no-no's I should probably add, but I'm thinking mainly of my own errors. Just baby yourself for a while…

    On our night staff is a gal who came in three times each night to play with Tom while I was In the hospital. She still empties his litter box at 11 PM each evening, and he jumps off the bed when he hears her open the door. And just down the hall is Tom's very best friend who took it upon herself to manage his food and water, rub his tummy, and generally keep him happy. She is 100 years old, and has a heart of pure gold! One of our maintenance men came in as often as he could to sit with Tom, and though my kitty is not a lap-sitter, I was surprised to learn he climbed up and had to be pushed off when work called. Another man I enlisted purposely, was a resident who had lost his cat just weeks before. It was not only a favor to me but a job he enjoyed at a time he was lonesome.

    So, you see, there are ways you can get necessities taken care of but allow people to enjoy your animals. Dogs need walks as well as food, and perhaps you have a friend who should walk but has no one to go with. Since your dog needs to get out, that may solve his or her problem.

I hope you have learned enough about colon cancer in my short book to help you keep from having the hardships many go through. And by knowing facts it's easier to help others. I wish you a happy and healthy life.
    Anne

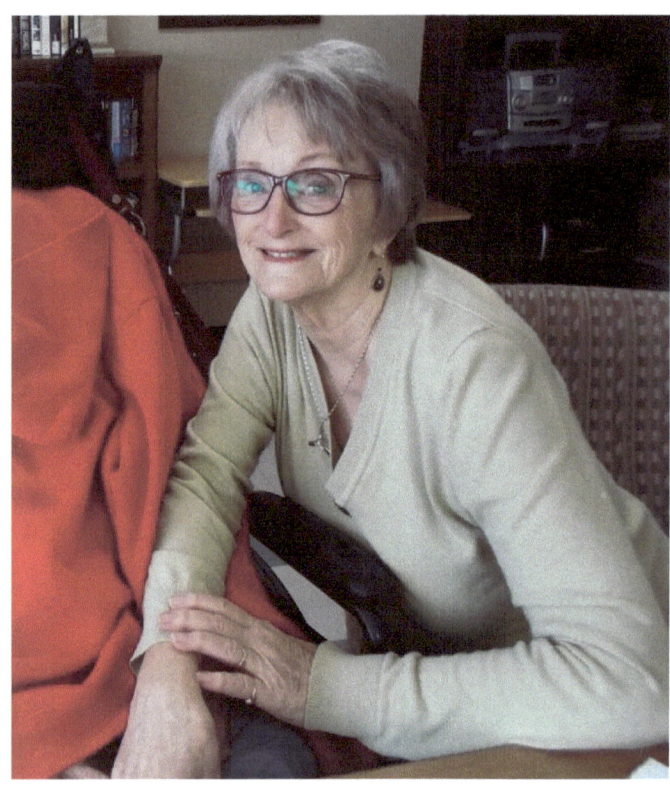